The Ideal Morning Routine

Lose Weight, Increase Productivity, Look Great

Ryder Management Inc.

Epigraph

"Feeling sorry for yourself and your present condition, is not only a waste of energy but the worst habit you could possibly have."

Dale Carnegie

"Habit, if not resisted, soon becomes necessity."

St. Augustine

.

Who is This Book For?

Are you feeling the effects of middle age?

Have you noticed that you are slowing down with any of your normal activities?

Are you worried about your health?

Do you pray for quality of life in your retirement years?

If you answered yes to any one of the above questions, then this book is for you.

Actually, The Ideal Morning Routine is recommended to anyone who is concerned with helping their body achieve its ideal weight and achieve ultimate health as well.

Each habit discussed in this book will help increase your productivity, boost your energy and help your body obtain its ideal weight. As you include more of the habits discussed in this book into your morning routine, each habit builds on the other and together, has a synergy effect that help achieve these goals faster. In other words, by starting each day with each habit is more powerful than any individual one on its own. BUT, and that's a big BUT, each individual habit is also quite powerful on its own.

You may find that some of the habits discussed will be easier to adopt for you than others will be. However, your goal is to include each and every one of these habits into your daily morning routine.

Once you have adopted all of these habits into your morning, you will feel and look on top of the world. At this point, you will be in a position to accomplish whatever you want.

Ryder Management Inc.

Table of Contents

Introduction

The intention of this book is to help you achieve your body's ideal weight and to help you achieve optimal health.

Any routine is made up of habits and there are 12 habits that make up the Ideal Morning Routine. It is necessary for you to adopt each one. Each one is discussed individually in the pages that follow. These 12 habits are designed to help you get the most out of your life, because life really is - short.

Although you can find a number of eBooks and blogs that discuss the habits of highly successful people, not one of them are "all inclusive" in containing all the habits discussed in this book.

Each of the habits contained in the Ideal Morning Routine will provide you with the maximum health and energy boosting benefits you can get. These benefits in turn help your body achieve and maintain its ideal weight and you to obtain optimal health.

Looking after your health should be your number one priority. Without our health our quality of life greatly deteriorates. You may not be able to fully appreciate the meaning in that statement unless you actually experienced (and heaven forbid) a loss of health.

Therefore, your personal priorities should include "me" time or at the very least, enough time for you to incorporate the Ideal Morning Routine into your life. By doing this for yourself, is an investment in your future. The habits that make up the Ideal Morning Routine discussed in this book will ensure that you remain strong so that you continue to be able to gain the most out of your life.

The Ideal Morning Routine is what brought me back from what I was told was a terminal liver disease. However, with shear and purposeful determination, I found my way back. In hindsight, I have learned never to take my health for granted again.

Ideal Morning Habit #1 - Get Up Earlier

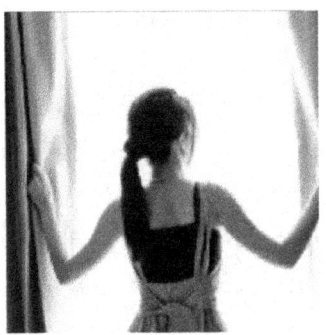

Get Up Earlier:

If your job is not a 9 to 5, do not worry or feel that waking up earlier does not apply to you. Even if you work afternoon or evening hours, the goal of getting up earlier is to help enable you to incorporate the Ideal Morning Routine into your morning because by doing so will change the quality of your life for the better. The objective of the Ideal Morning Routine is to help your body achieve its ideal weight; increase your energy and therefore your productivity along with your health and quality of life too.

To Do:

At the beginning, you will need to get up at least one to two hours earlier if you are presently rushed out the door upon rising in the morning. Allow me to impress on you that the benefits of incorporating the 12 Ideal Morning Habits discussed in this book into your life is to change your life for the better. Upon incorporating these habits, you will feel more enjoyment from life, like never before. The key, remember, is to adopt all of the habits into your morning routine.

More Information:

If you start each day by incorporating as many of the habits discussed in this book into your morning as you can, I can guarantee you that your life will change for the better. Not only will you start feeling better, you will benefit from increased energy and health. Lacking energy is the number one killer to quality of life. Gaining more energy will benefit you in so many aspects of your life that you will not want to overlook any one of the Ideal Morning Habits from your routine. Therefore, your goal of getting up earlier is to ensure that you make the time for the Ideal Morning Routine in its entirety.

New research has shown that "while sunlight can reset our circadian clocks, our bodies also depend on internal timekeeping devices or "endogenous clocks" ...to maintain Ideal health" http://onforb.es/1cc5fX3 . As an aside, circadian rhythm is any biological process that displays endogenous, entrainable (brought into rhythm) oscillation of about 24 hours. These 24 hour rhythms are driven by a circadian clock, and they have been widely observed in plants, animals, fungi and cyanobacteria. From widipedia.org

This study shows that the best thing that you can do for your body and health is to develop a routine that is consistent within a 24 hour period. In other words, if you are unable to develop a consistent routine following the suns orbit, as long as your routine is consistent within a 24 hour period, you will still help your body the best. In this way, your body can rely on a steady routine for it to perform in ultimate health.

How You Will Benefit:

By waking up at the same time every day, regardless of the time of day, your body will become regulated to fall asleep according to the set routine or schedule. The advantages continue because soon, your body will be accustomed to waking up at the new time, making it easier for you to get out of bed. By waking up earlier to invest in your health by completing this Ideal Morning Routine will also make you less stressed at the start of your day. You are less stressed because you won't be in a rush to get out the door. Therefore, unnecessary stress, tension and the feeling of being rushed can be avoided.

Ideal Morning Habit #2 – Oil Pulling

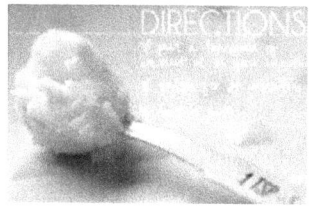

Oil Pulling:

You may have heard of the age old ancient practice of oil pulling. If you have wondered what all the hoopla was or is all about, let me assure you, I can personally attest to this daily practice. This ultimate morning habit will capitulate, you to better health and better looks almost instantly.

To Do:

Upon rising each morning, before you do anything else, scoop up to one teaspoon of high quality oil, such as extra virgin coconut oil or organic hemp oil and place in your mouth. Using saliva in your mouth, swish the oil all around your mouth and between your teeth. Do this for approximately 5 to 20 minutes. If you are not able to swish for the full 20 minutes, don't worry. I can assure you that by doing this age old practice for at least five minutes every day will still bring you big results.

After you have finished swishing this oil in your mouth, spit the oil out into the garbage to avoid clogged sinks.

Once you have spit the oil out, rinse and gargle with warm salted water (add up to ¼ teaspoon of salt to ½ cup of warm water). This ensures that you have rid your mouth of all the oil filled bacteria in your mouth. After you have rinsed your mouth, you are ready to brush and floss as normal.

Oil pulling can also be performed in the evening, following the procedure, to gain added health benefits faster.

More Information:

Oil pulling is an ancient Ayurvedic technique that involves swishing as much as one tablespoon of high quality oil (such as coconut oil or hemp oil) in your mouth, first thing in the morning, for approximately 5 to 20 minutes before spitting it out. It is important NOT to swallow this oil as it will contain a host of toxins and bacteria that it accumulated and that accumulated in your mouth overnight.

Oil pulling is most effective first thing in the morning, before putting anything else into your mouth. In the Ayurvedic text Charka Samhita, oil pulling is said to cure over 30 systemic diseases ranging from headaches, migraines, diabetes, and toxicity in the body. In addition, this practice has unbelievable oral health benefits including strengthening and whitening your teeth; preventing tooth decay, gum disease, cracked lips and more.

Oil pulling is recognized in Complementary and Alternative Medicine (CAM) as a preventative and curative healing remedy. Oil pulling is found to also benefit the kidneys, lungs, liver, heart, and digestive system.

After swishing approximately 1 teaspoon to 1 tablespoon of high quality oil for up to 20 minutes in your mouth and between your teeth, spit the oil out in the garbage. It is advisable not to spit this oil out in your sink or toilet due to the extra cleaning it will cause, not to mention the possibility of clogged drains. The benefits you will gain by performing this single action far out way any nuisance you may think this action has.

How You Will Benefit:

You will benefit immediately with oil pulling. To begin, you will feel more energy almost immediately. By removing all the bacteria and toxins from your mouth that have developed overnight will also leave you with fresher breath and very soon, whiter teeth.

Ideal Morning Habit #3 - Drink a Glass of Lemon Water

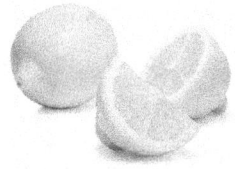

Drink a glass of warm lemon water:

Fresh lemons are one of nature's best remedies that can combat a variety of illnesses and the liver is one of the biggest benefactors. By consuming a glass of lemon water first thing in the morning will help activate your system.

To Do:

After your oil pull and once you have cleaned your teeth by brushing with coconut oil, squeeze the juice of half a lemon into a glass of room temperature filtered water and drink down.

More Information:

The list of benefits of drinking lemon water in the morning is long and includes:

Lemon water provides your body with electrolytes which help to hydrate your body.

Lemon juice is similar in atomic structure to the stomach's digestive juices. Therefore, drinking lemon water has a positive effect on our gastrointestinal tract and it helps to cleanse the bowel by flushing out waste more efficiently. Since lemons contain citric acid, this interacts with other enzymes and acids which make it easier to stimulate the secretion of gastric juice, which aids healthy digestion.

Our liver produces more enzymes with the aid of lemon water than from any other food or beverage. Lemon water also cleanses the liver and stimulates it into releasing toxins. It also helps regulate natural bowel movements. With less toxins circulating in our body, you can expect clearer skin that naturally glows.

Since lemons are also rich in Vitamin C, drinking lemon water helps boost our immune system and helps to fight off colds and flus. Lemons are also powerful antioxidants and protect our bodies from free radicals; this further boosts our immune system.

Lemons are also a great anti-aging remedy. The antioxidant properties in lemons help fight free radical damage. Free radical damage is what speeds up the aging process. Also, since lemons are rich in Vitamin C, this helps create collagen and keep wrinkles at bay.

Lemons contain a high content of potassium which helps our nervous system to function properly. Since low levels of potassium have been linked to depression and anxiety, drinking lemon water will help keep these conditions at bay.

Lemons contain pectin, a soluble fiber that is commonly found in citrus fruits as well as apples. Pectin is known to reduce hunger since fiber creates a feeling of fullness. By feeling full longer, you are more likely to make healthy food choices.

Lemons are one of the most alkalizing foods for the body and helps balance pH levels. A balanced pH level in the body is important in the prevention of cancer and other diseases.

Lemon juice is a natural diuretic and encourages the production of urine. This helps relieve bloating and swelling in the body.

Lemon water helps reduce pain and inflammation in joints and knees since it dissolves uric acid.

How You Will Benefit:

By starting your day with lemon water, you benefit by the increased vitamins that lemons contain. Lemons also help to get your system moving and helps eliminate toxins from your body. This benefits you by providing you with more energy.

Ideal Morning Habit #4 – Take Chlorella

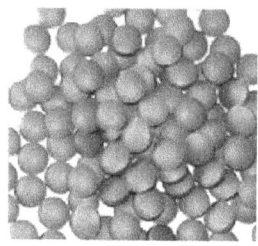

Take chlorella tablets in place of a vitamin tablet:

Chlorella contains more chlorophyll than any other plant on earth. Chlorophyll improves immunity, alkalinity and inflammation. It is rich in a number of vitamins, discussed below and is widely known for its ability to bind with toxins and chemicals in the body.

To Do:

Chlorella offers more benefits than a single multivitamin tablet. In this regard, there is no need to take both Chlorella and a multivitamin tablet. Instead, substitute chlorella tablets in place of your daily multivitamin tablet to gain more than what your single multivitamin tablet offers.

More Information:

Chlorella is widely known as a powerful "superfood" supplement that contains a high amount of nutrients. Chlorella is single celled, water grown micro algae that contains Vitamins A, C, E and K. It is also one of the few whole food sources of vitamin D and contains the entire Vitamin B complex. In addition, chlorella contains beta-carotene, magnesium, iron, potassium, phosphorous, zinc and calcium. Chlorella is also a rich source of protein with a balance of all the essential amino acids, essential fatty acids including gamma linolenic acid (GLA). As already mentioned chlorella is widely known for its ability to bind with toxins and chemicals in the body as well as aiding in digestion and fighting candida.

Many people have reported increased energy and elevated moods from taking chlorella. Since chlorella is also rich in carotenoids, which prevent oxidation, chlorella is also known for its remarkable cancer-fighting benefits. Studies also show that chlorella can increase levels of HDL and reduce your body's fat percentage as well as improve insulin sensitivity and help to balance blood sugar levels over time.

Chlorella is available in tablet and powder forms.

In terms of multivitamin tablets, in December of 2013, WebMD cited three new studies that found that multivitamins did not improve health. Although the multivitamin industry is a multibillion dollar industry in the US, growing evidence suggests that multivitamins offer little or nothing in the way of health benefits. http://www.webmd.com/vitamins-and-supplements/news/20131216/experts-dont-waste-your-money-on-multivitamins

How You Will Benefit:

Chlorella is an all-natural supplement that boosts your energy, supports fat loss and helps detox heavy metals such as mercury and lead from your body.

Studies show that Chlorella benefits your entire body by supporting healthy hormonal function, good cardiovascular health, lowers blood pressure and cholesterol and aids in our body's detoxification.

Chlorella is ranked as one of the top ten health foods in the world when comparing its' nutrient density score. Moreover, on a gram for gram basis Chlorella is more significantly dense than other green vegetables including broccoli, spinach and even kale.

The biggest benefits offered by Chlorella include helps regulate hormones, helps with metabolism, improves circulation and promotes higher energy levels. It also helps to reduce weight and body fat, and removes stored toxins.

Ideal Morning Habit #5 – ACV

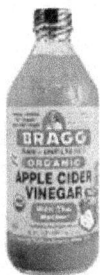

Apple Cider Vinegar (ACV):

Drinking warm water with up to a teaspoon (tsp) of raw organic apple cider vinegar in the morning will increase your health and stamina immensely.

To Do:

To start, add ½ tsp of raw organic apple cider vinegar (ACV) to a small glass of warm water and drink up. For added benefit, mix in ½ tsp of raw organic honey too. Once you have become used to ACV, increase the amount to 1 teaspoon (tsp) in a larger glass of water.

You always want to be sure to dilute ACV in water.

More Information:

Diluted raw apple cider vinegar (ACV) has been used throughout history to treat a wide range of health ailments. Over the centuries, it was one of the most traditional cures for almost anything. In addition, ACV adds a number of health benefits to your body including assistance with achieving your ideal weight. ACV has anti-bacterial, anti-fungal and anti-viral properties thus making it an effective health remedy against a number of diseases, illness and ailments.

Hippocrates, the ancient Greek physician, was a proponent of apple cider vinegar and was known to treat his patients suffering from digestive issues with it. The feared Japanese samurai warriors relied upon ACV to maintain their strength. ACV was used by Ancient Persians to prevent the accumulation of fatty tissues in the body. In addition, during the US Civil War and World War I, it was used in the US to treat wounds on the battle field.

The benefits of consuming ACV include:

ACV contains potassium and enzymes which help banish fatigue. In addition, the amino acids found in ACV help prevent a build-up of lactic acid in our body which helps to further ward off fatigue.

ACV will balance your body's pH level: Even though ACV is acidic, it has an alkaline effect in our body, thus balancing our body's pH level. By causing the pH levels in our body to become more alkaline, ACV is able to help prevent cancer.

ACV will help you detox: Due to the toxins we are faced with on a daily basis, it is important to detox. Detoxification is a process whereby harmful toxins are eliminated from our bodies which then allows our organs to work properly.

ACV boosts metabolism which can aid in weight loss. In addition, due to the acetic acid level in ACV, helps you to feel full longer.

ACV can help reduce and eliminate heartburn: Acid reflux is caused by having too little acid in your stomach. Consuming ACV rectifies this condition and even helps to soothe intestinal spasms.

It is recommended that you only consume raw organic apple cider vinegar. Raw ACV is unpasteurized and therefore does not contain any added chemicals nor has it been stripped of its natural benefits. ACV that looks plain and clear has been processed and it is advised to avoid this type completely.

Unpasteurized or organic ACV contains mother of vinegar, which has a cobweb like appearance and makes the vinegar appear cloudy. This is the only way ACV should be consumed.

How You Will Benefit:

In a study published on PubMed, research showed that acetic acid, a main component of vinegar, was found to suppress body fat accumulation. http://www.ncbi.nlm.nih.gov/pubmed/19661687

This study showed a decrease in belly fat with continual consumption of ACV.

Acetic acid, a component of ACV, is also a potent antimicrobial, capable of defending against, bacteria, viruses, fungus and other microorganisms. This ability supports your autoimmune defense.

Ideal Morning Habit #6 – Morning Walk

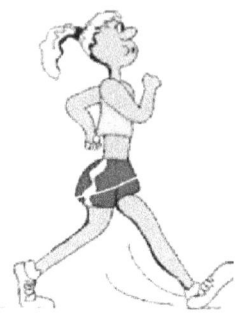

Morning Walk:

Start your day with a brisk morning walk. Even a stroll around the block, to begin, has many health benefits for you to reap. Beginning your day with physical activity ensures that you have mental sharpness for the rest of your day.

To Do:

After your oil pull, lemon water, ACV water and chlorella tablets, put on your walking shoes, it's time for fresh air and a brisk stroll around the block. If you are just starting out, even a walk of less than 20 minutes will invigorate you for the rest of your day.

Before you begin it is necessary to perform some stretching exercises. In addition, once you have completed your morning walk, you are encouraged to perform additional stretching exercises. By doing this, you will help your muscles become accustomed to this new routine.

More Information:

Modern research has shown that a brisk morning walk on a daily basis will benefit you in so many ways. Regardless of your age, sex and physical ability, walking can reduce your risk of chronic disease, boost your self-esteem and help you obtain ideal health and your body's ideal weight, thus enabling you to get the most out of your life.

The Department of Health and Human Services advises that healthy individuals include a form of aerobic exercise and strength training into their daily fitness plans. More specifically, they recommend at least 150 minutes of moderate aerobic activity each week. This translates into 20 minutes of daily activity such as walking.

Walking does not require any special equipment other than a good pair of walking shoes. Walking does not entail driving anywhere to begin, since you can reap the benefits of walking as soon as you step outside.

How You Will Benefit:

The benefits of a morning walk, apart from physical benefits such as becoming more toned, you will also experience mental benefits. Almost immediately, you should start to feel less stress as tension is released through this morning activity. This in turn will have the effect of a happier mood which in itself brings the benefit of making you look amazing.

Ideal Morning Habit #7 – Stretching

Stretching:

After your morning walk and walk cool down, it is necessary to stretch certain muscles in your body to avoid soreness or muscle stiffness. Stretching is an important and powerful part of any exercise program, including walking.

To Do:

Repeat each of the following stretches on each leg, holding for a count of 15-30 seconds:

Quad Stretch:

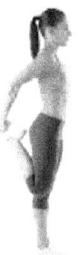

For the quad stretch, pictured above, you may want to use a wall, fence or post to help with balance and stability. Since the quadriceps muscles are used in walking, it is necessary to stretch these muscles after your walk to prevent soreness. To begin, stand erect and bend your knee behind you so that you can grasp your foot from behind and hold your heel against your butt. Hold this position for 15-30 seconds before releasing your foot. Stand on both feet and then repeat this stretch with your opposite foot.

Hip-flexor Stretch:

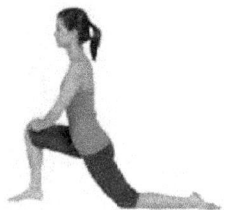

To stretch the right hip flexors, kneel on your right knee and put your left foot in front of you. Your left hip and knee should be about 90 degrees. If you find this position, pictured above, uncomfortable, consider putting a cushion on the floor, under your knee. Keep your chest up and be sure not to bend forward at the hips. Hold this position for 15-30 seconds and then stand on both feet before switching to your left hip flexors. Repeat.

Hamstring Stretch:

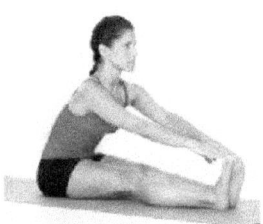

Hamstrings are very strong muscles and may take months of stretching to get them to a reasonably flexible level. Therefore, please do not expect any quick results.

To begin stretching your hammies, sit on the floor with your legs straight in front of you. Sit up straight and breathe in. Breathe out and bend at your hips reaching forward to touch your toes. Make sure that your toes are pointing up. Hold this forward stretch for 15-30 seconds as you feel the stretch in your hamstrings. Return to sitting up straight. Repeat this exercise.

Butterfly/groin Stretch:

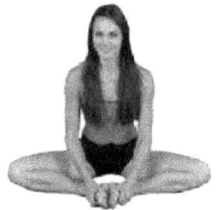

Sit on the floor with your knees bent and your feet pulled together so that your legs are in the butterfly position, pictured above. Put your hands around your ankles. Keeping your spine straight and your butt pressed into the floor, slowly bend forward at the waist. Using your elbows, carefully press them against your knees, gently pushing them apart. It is important not to round your back. Hold this position for 15-30 seconds before relaxing. Repeat up to three times

Calf-Stretch:

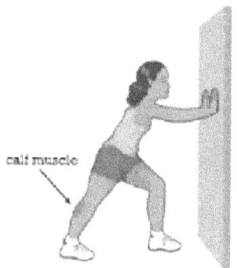

calf muscle

The calf muscle actually consists of two muscles: the gastrocnemius and the deeper muscle called the soleus. Both of these insert into the Achilles tendon located at the back of your ankle. Since the gastrocnemius originates from above your knee, in order to stretch it, the knee must be fully extended. Since the soleus muscle originates below the knee, the knee need not be extended in order to stretch this muscle.

Stand away from the wall and put your right foot behind you ensuring your toes are facing the wall. Keeping your heel on the ground, lean forward with your right knee straight and hold this position for 30 seconds. Return to standing position and repeat with your left leg.

Stand away from the wall and put your right foot behind you ensuring your toes are facing the wall. Lean forward at the ankle while bending your right knee, keeping your heel on the ground. Hold this position for 30 seconds. Return to standing position and repeat with your left leg.

More Information:

Stretching is an important and powerful part of any exercise program, including walking. Most aerobic and strength training exercises, such as walking, inherently cause muscles to contract and tighten, causing sore and aching muscles. Stretching your muscles after your walking routine is important to prevent them from becoming stiff and sore.

Stretching your muscles after your walk will help improve the range of motion in your joints, increase blood circulation and help to prevent sore muscles.

As in most things, it is necessary to know and become familiar with certain rules so that you gain the most from your new walking routine. To begin with, it is important to remember to never stretch cold muscles. The best time to stretch your muscles is after your walk or during your walk, once you have warmed up. However, if you know you have problem areas in your body, these areas can be stretched prior to beginning your walk.

The best warm-up exercise for your walk is to start with a five (5) minute walking warm-up. Start by walking at a medium pace and then slowly increase your pace so that by the end of the five minutes, you can easily begin your walking routine by continuing into it.

Stretching your muscles after you exercise can help you to increase the range of motion in your joints. Remember to begin your stretch slowly and hold it gently. Only stretch to the point of feeling a gentle pull, but never to the point of pain. If you do feel pain, you have gone too far. Forget "No Pain No Gain"; it does not apply to us in our walking routine.

When you are stretching, keep it gentle; breathe freely while holding your stretch; hold each stretch for 20 to 30 seconds, and then release. If you have any problems with a stretch, hold for a lesser time and then repeat the stretch. To begin, each stretch should be done once if holding for thirty seconds, or twice if holding for a count of 15 seconds. Seniors will benefit by working up to a count of 60 seconds per stretch.

How You Will Benefit:

In addition to the above stretching exercises that focus on preventing your leg muscles from becoming sore and or stiff, you can also touch your toes by standing straight with your feet shoulder distance apart and stretch to the ceiling, before bobbing to touch the floor. This stretching exercise ensures that your back muscles are stretched, thus preventing unnecessary back pain.

Performing the above stretching exercises will ensure that your leg and back muscles remain flexible and prevent stiffness and soreness from your morning walk. Stretching after your walk will also ensure that your morning walk remains enjoyable.

Ideal Morning Habit #8 – Cold Shower

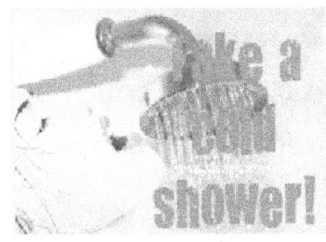

Cold Shower:

Did you know that cold showers can improve blood circulation, help boost white blood cell activity, dissolve tension, balance hormones, improve circulation and help your body detox?

To Do:

After you have cooled down from your exercise, walk or run, you are ready to jump in the shower. Although you may not be thrilled with the idea of only a cold shower, by at least rinsing with cold water prior to getting out of the shower can still bring you the cold water benefits. Therefore, Ideal Morning Habit #6 is to end your shower with a cold water rinse for as long as you can. In addition to the health benefits it brings you, it will also greatly reduce the chance of mold from forming in your shower.

More Information:

You may be surprised to learn that cold showers provide a number of mental, psychological and overall health benefits. Exposure to cold water provides a boost to our immune system which reduces the risk of illness. Since a cold shower increases your heart rate and speeds up blood circulation, the result is increased energy. In addition, cold shower promote healthier hair and adds a glow to your skin since cold water closes the pores in your skin, locking in natural oils keeping toxins out.

After you shower normally, gradually decrease the temperature until you have reached full cold. Do not stand under the cold water for longer than ten minutes.

Ending your shower with cold water also removes the steam build up in the shower and bathroom, reducing the likelihood of mold from developing.

How You Will Benefit:

Be ending your shower with cold water, may sound daunting at first but consider the following benefits:

Increased alertness: The shock of cold water on our body actually has the ability of increasing our body temperature thus keeping us warm internally. The cold water triggers our overall oxygen intake; increases our heart which also increases our blood circulation thus giving us a natural dose of energy for the day.

Eases stress: Having a cold shower has been shown to increase the production of glutathione, an antioxidant that keeps all other antioxidants performing at their optimal level.

Stimulates weigh loss: Cold showers can have an unexpected benefit of stimulating weight loss in your body. Our bodies contain two types of fat, white and brown fat. Brown fat is the good fat and generates heat that keeps our bodies warm. This fat is activated when exposed to extreme cold, according to the Harvard Medical School.

Ideal Morning Habit #9 – Hemp Breakfast

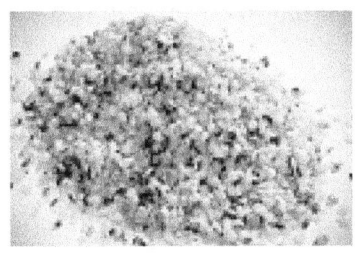

Eat a Healthy Hemp Breakfast:

Did you know that raw shelled hemp seeds are one of nature's perfect foods, a superfood? Hemp provides a broad spectrum of health benefits including the promotion of weight loss, increased and sustained energy, rapid recovery from disease and injury, lowered cholesterol and blood pressure, reduced inflammation, improved circulation and an improved immune system.

To Do:

Make a satisfying Hemp Smoothie to start your day:

Ingredients:

5 Tbsps. of raw shelled organic hemp seed

½ cup of frozen blueberries

1 small ripe banana

1 ½ cup of filtered water

Directions:

In your high speed blender or NutriBullet, add all ingredients and then blend until smooth.

Enjoy!

Options:

Add ½ tsp of cinnamon, nutmeg, turmeric, ginger or any spice of your choice.

More Information:

Hemp seeds are one of the most nutritious seeds on the planet and offer a very wide range of health benefits, compared to other nuts and seeds.

Hemp seed has a balanced ratio of Omega-6 and Omega-3 essential fatty acids, along with GLA, protein, Vitamins A, B, E and D. Hemp is also rich in sodium, calcium, iron and dietary fiber thus being able to provide you with most of your dietary needs for optimal health.

Hemp is a natural appetite suppressant and is able to help induce weight loss because consuming them, makes you feel full longer. Studies show that by adding just four to five tablespoons (Tbsps.) of hemp seed to your morning meal can reduce your food cravings significantly longer. In addition, hemp boosts your energy level helping you to be more productive during your day.

Research shows that hemp is an excellent source of protein containing 10 essential amino acids, healthy polyunsaturated fats most notably the Essential Fatty Acids (EFA) Omega-6 arranged in perfect balance with Omega 3 (4:1) for our body's Ideal needs. Hemp milk, made easily from hemp seed, does not need to be fortified or enriched to bring it up to optimal nutritional value for our body.

Hemp is a food and textile crop containing fiber and seeds. Due to its distant relationship to marijuana, growing the hemp plant has been forbidden in the US since the introduction of the Marijuana Stamp Act near the beginning of the twentieth century.

Since hemp contains only trace amounts of THC, it that, the popular phrase about hemp seeds is that "you can't get high on the seeds, you can only get healthy."

Hemp's use as an agriculture crop dates back over 10,000 years where it was cultivated in China, even before the soy bean.

Hemp has a very long and interesting history; however, the focus of our discussion is on the multitude of health benefits it offers.

How You Will Benefit:

Hemp seeds are a concentrated source of essential fats, complete proteins, enzymes and vitamins.

Essential Fatty Acids (EFA):

Hemp seeds are low in saturated fats and are promoted by many health practitioners as the perfect food for the human diet. In the book "Fats that Heal, Fats that Kill", the author provides evidence that the oil in the hemp seed is the best source of EFA of any food. The hemp seed contain one of the highest sources of Omega-6 and Omega-3 EFA in a perfect balanced ratio of 4:1.

Essential fatty acids are called essential to our diet because they play many important roles in our body. EFA are necessary for neurological functioning, the stability of cell membranes, and the transfer of oxygen, inflammatory regulation, immune response and the maintenance of cardiovascular health.

Hemp seeds also contain GLA or gamma linolenic acid, another important EFA that is somewhat rare. GLA is known to reduce inflammation, help with eczema as well as decrease breast tenderness in women. GLA is especially concentrated in hemp seed oil as well as in evening primrose oil and borage oil.

Hemp seeds also contain a high amount of Vitamin E, an important antioxidant that inhibits the oxidation of other molecules in the body.

Hemp seed is also considered a heart healthy fat source that can help reduce inflammation, blood cholesterol levels along with high blood pressure associated with cardiovascular disease.

Weight-loss:

The nutritional density and the soluble fiber content found in hemp seeds are especially important for losing or controlling weight. Hemp seeds can provide a source of long lasting fuel that can satisfy your appetite over a long period of time.

Because hemp seeds are also very high in protein, they are the perfect food for those wanting to replace dairy and animal products in their diet and follow a more plant based diet.

The hemp seed contains all the amino acids and are a highly digestible, complete source of protein. Hemp seeds contain 66% edestin and 33% albumin globulin proteins. Edestin is considered a very digestible form of protein that is found exclusively unique to the hemp seeds. Hemp also does not contain any enzyme inhibitors such as that found in soy or whey powder. Enzyme inhibitors can prevent the absorption of nutrients.

Since hemp seeds do not contain phytic acid or enzyme inhibitors, they do not need to be soaked and rinsed first, like other nuts, before consuming.

Ideal Morning Habit #10 – Tulsi Holy Basil Tea

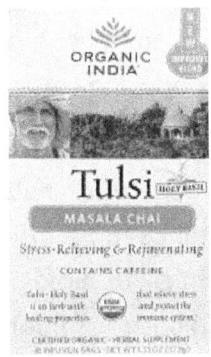

Drink a cup of Holy Basil (Tulsi) tea:

Holy Basil functions as an adaptogen, enhancing the body's natural response to physical and emotional stress by helping it function optimally during stressful times. It has a long tradition of medicinal use in Ayurvedic medicine and has an amazing number of health benefits.

Holy Basil (Ocimum sanctum) is not the same as the pesto or sweet variety of basil (Ocimum basilicum) used in cooking spaghetti sauce.

To Do:

Enjoy a cup of Holy Basil tea. This tea rivals the health benefits found in green tea alone. Holy Basil tea is sold in combination with other herbs as well as in combination with green tea.

Holy Basil Tea or Tulsi tea is a caffeine free herbal tea that has strong antibacterial and antiviral properties. In addition, it has powerful antioxidants that help strengthen your immune system.

More Information:

For over 5,000 years, Holy Basil, also known as Tulsi or Tulsi Holy Basil, has been considered India's "Queen of Herb" and has long been considered sacred. It has a history of being revered as a healing balm for mind, body and spirit.

Modern research has classified Tulsi Holy Basil as an adaptogenic herb. Adaptogens are natural substances that help the body increase resistance to harmful factors such as stressors of various physical, chemical or biological causes. Adaptogenic herbs have been used in both Traditional Chinese Medicine (TCM) and Ayurvedic medicine for thousands of years as a way of promoting and maintaining health. Many adaptogenic herbs are also referred to as rejuvenative herbs, qi tonic herbs, rasayanas and restorative herbs. These herbs help the body adapt to their environment and the physical and emotional stressors found there. They also help the body support normal functions and restores balance in the body.

The Tulsi or holy basil plant is known to have many medicinal properties. The leaves are also a known nerve tonic (also called nervine), which helps calm and the nervous system, in addition to being considered an adaptogenic herb. The leaves are also known to sharpen memory thus making them an effective remedy against Alzheimer's disease.

How You Will Benefit:

Thousands of people attribute their ability to handle stress relatively easily is due to their regular consumption of Holy Basil or Tulsi Tea. Tulsi is described as a healing herb that fights stress. The taste and scent of Tulsi tea itself, is soothing and relaxing.

Since Tulsi Holy Basil is considered an adaptogen, it is therefore an herbal that supports a systematic resistance to stress and stressors with a normalizing effect on the body.

Since Tulsi tea offers so many benefits, you will benefit in so many ways once you incorporate this adaptogenic herbal tea into your daily diet.

Ideal Morning Habit #11 – Plan Your Day

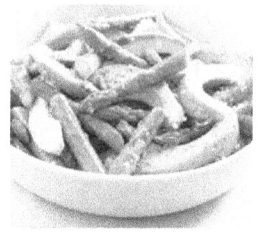

Plan Your Day's Snacks and Meals:

One of the first things in planning your day is to plan your snacks and meals for the day. This is important for your Ideal health because, as Benjamin Franklin said, "If you fail to plan, you are planning to fail."

Do you need to stop at the Market or Grocery Store and pick up some produce for the day? Do you have everything you need at home to enable you to pack your lunch (and snacks)?

To Do:

Since you are what you eat, it is important to plan how you are going to take your snacks, drinks and lunch to work with you. Do you have a stressful job? Do you find that you get stressed during your day? If this is the case, plan to pack specific herbal tea; herbs that are known as adaptogens such as Holy Basil Tea, Lavender Tea, Passionflower Tea or Rooibos (pronounced Roy Boss) Tea, to name a few.

Are you able to purchase a fresh avocado salad at lunch a reasonable amount? You can always bring the protein for topping. This adds to your salad's health benefits plus saves you money. Toppings for your salad, such as protein, to buy in advance includes things such as, sunflower seed, shelled walnuts, cashews or almonds, and of course, hemp seed. Remember that you don't have to spend a lot of money to get the Ideal health from your food.

Consider packing snacks such as shelled walnuts, almonds or cashews; fruit such as apples, banana, grapes; vegetables such as sliced carrots, celery, cucumbers, broccoli etc. You are only limited by your imagination and what your market or grocery store carries.

More Information:

By planning to ensure you have on hand throughout your day, healthy snacks, adaptogenic tea and water enables you to make the most out of your day. This type of planning also ensures that you do not have to rely on less than optimal choices for mid-morning or mid-afternoon snacks.

How You Will Benefit:

By planning what you will eat and snack on while you are at work, you are ensuring that you don't have to buy junk food, processed food and food that will not be benefiting you the most. By adhering to a planned food and snacking diet, you are committing to healthy eating and healthy snacks. In this way too, you are able to avoid low blood sugar levels thus keeping your energy and productivity up.

Resisting the urge to reach for candy, chips or even fast food such as burgers when you are hit with a snack attack will make a big difference in your health and waistline, regardless of your age. Through planning too, you are able to avoid any periods of extreme hunger since you have on hand quick and easy snacks such as fruit, vegetables, nuts or dried fruit.

Nutrition is the key to a healthy lifestyle and a healthy life.

Ideal Morning Habit #12 – Deep Breathing

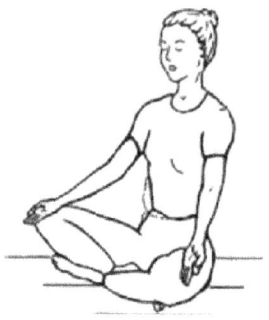

Simple Deep Breathing Exercises:

Practicing regular, mindful breathing can be energizing, calming and helpful at controlling stress and even your weight. Deep breathing, since it is something we are able to control and regulate, is also useful for achieving a clear state of mind. It is particularly beneficial before leaving for work.

To Do:

The most basic thing to remember when practicing deep breathing is that your breath begins upon a full exhale since you can't inhale fully unless your lungs are completely empty. It is also important to remember to breathe in through your nose.

To begin, sit in a comfortable position with your hands on your knees. You can sit you're your legs crossed on the floor or sit upright in a chair.

With your shoulders relaxed, start by exhaling fully through your nose, counting to five. While exhaling and counting to five, draw your diaphragm in to help deflate your lungs.

Inhale slowly through your nose while counting to five. Expand your stomach as you breathe in.

Close your eyes and repeat five to ten times.

More Information:

Simple breathing exercises can have a profound effect on your health and life. Many Eastern Practitioners have long recognized the importance of breathing in cultivating a positive relationship between mind and body. It has been reported too that Asian women report fewer menopausal symptoms such as hot flashes, as a result of their routine practice of deep breathing.

How You Will Benefit:

Deep breathing can improve your lymph system cleansing. The expansion and contraction of your diaphragm stimulates your lymphatic system and also massages your internal organs. This helps the body rid itself of toxins, leaving more room in your cells for an optimal exchange of oxygen.

Deep breathing contains many of the benefits of physical exercise, including helping your body lose excess weight. Although not a substitute for exercise, deep breathing is also an excellent first step for anyone beginning an exercise program because deep breathing enhances the benefits of all forms of exercise.

So many times, we take time for others without taking any time for ourselves. We will rise to the demand of looking after the basic needs of others but not our own.

Taking the time to breathe more fully and deeply is a very small but vital way to do something extremely important for ourselves. By paying consciously controlling our inhalation and our exhalation will slowly but surely move us towards a healthier and happier life.

Tips, Tricks and Trivia

Once you have included each habit described in this book, you can save time by combining one or two of the activities. For example, you can combine lemon water with your ACV distilled water, if you desire.

Consider also combining your Holy Basil tea with planning your day, to save additional time.

The important point with the Ideal Morning Routine is NOT to eliminate any step.

Did you know that walking is considered the #1 "Participation Sport" on the planet? During the work week, due to time constraints, you may not have time to meet with a walking club. However, on week-ends you may want to consider joining a walking club as a way to become more committed to walking. Walking clubs can provide additional benefits including meeting new friends.

When choosing good quality oil for oil pulling, consider using Extra Virgin Coconut Oil. Not only is this oil NOT refined, it tastes absolutely wonderful.

There are only two broad categories of coconut oil being sold on the market today. These two categories can be described as refined as in those that are produced at an industrial level and those that start fresh and need much less refining. The latter group is called raw or virgin coconut oil.

When choosing good quality apple cider vinegar, consider using Braggs Apple Cider Vinegar (ACV).

Replace table salt with Himalayan Pink Salt (HPS). Table salt has been processed to the point of having any nutrients removed whereas Himalayan Pink Salt is the purest salt on earth. Some experts are now hinting that table salt may actually be bad for your health.

Eliminate wheat and dairy from your diet.

Eliminate or greatly cut down on consuming junk food.

Flood your gut with good bacteria.

Closing Remarks

The purpose of this book is to help ensure you are able to get the most out of your life. In order to achieve this goal, your health must be your number one priority.

Whether you are in your 40's, 50's, 60's or older, at some point you will begin to feel the effects of advancing age. The only person, who should be in charge of your own individual health, is You. In this regard, it is important to take steps to increase your health.

Although I hope it is different for you, for me, every doctor and specialist I met during the most scary health ordeal I had to go through, told me not to waste my time or money on "quackery" cures. This was the response in reply to my questions involving any natural health product, including some discussed in this book. Since I flat out refused to believe these allopathic specialists' opinion, I took it upon myself to consult those practitioners skilled in Ayurvedic, Ancient Chinese Medicine and Native North American medicine who all believe in natural remedies, remedies that have been passed down through hundreds of years of practice.

I sincerely hope that you adopt the Ideal Morning Routine discussed in this book because it will help your body to achieve its ideal weight and help you obtain optimal health.

References and Resources

Healing Source: http://www.healing-source.com/about_HempFoods.htm

World's Healthiest Foods:
http://www.whfoods.com/genpage.php?tname=foodspice&dbid=27

Natural News: http://www.naturalnews.com/hemp.html

Healing the Body:

http://www.healingthebody.ca/healing-benefits-of-chlorella/

All about Coconut Oil: http://coconutoil.com/

ABOUT THE AUTHOR

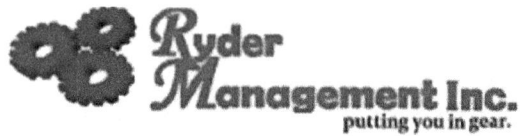

Based in London Ontario Canada, Ryder Management Inc is an umbrella organization that brings together likeminded individuals who are concerned with helping others. Ryder Management Inc's main concerns include the truth about health, cancer and medical cannabis.

Contact us through email at *info@RyderManagement.ca*

and ask to be notified of upcoming free Kindle books.

Visit our Amazon Author page where you will find a complete list of over 25 book titles at:

http://www.amazon.com/Ryder-Management-Inc/e/B00ICGMCRS

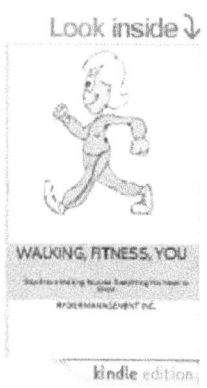

The Ideal Morning Routine

www.ingramcontent.com/pod-product-compliance
Lightning Source LLC
Chambersburg PA
CBHW070837290526
45795CB00002B/893